T0197132

Granny's
REVELATION

QUIT BLOWING SMOKE
IN ONE DAY

RICHARD H. BOBO

authorHOUSE®

AuthorHouse™
1663 Liberty Drive
Bloomington, IN 47403
www.authorhouse.com
Phone: 1 (800) 839-8640

Published by AuthorHouse   09/16/2015

ISBN: 978-1-5049-2465-8 (sc)
ISBN: 978-1-5049-2466-5 (hc)
ISBN: 978-1-5049-2464-1 (e)

Library of Congress Control Number: 2015911848

Print information available on the last page.

Any people depicted in stock imagery provided by Thinkstock are models,
and such images are being used for illustrative purposes only.
Certain stock imagery © Thinkstock.

This book is printed on acid-free paper.

Because of the dynamic nature of the Internet, any web addresses or
links contained in this book may have changed since publication and
may no longer be valid. The views expressed in this work are solely those
of the author and do not necessarily reflect the views of the publisher,
and the publisher hereby disclaims any responsibility for them.

Dedication

This book is dedicated to Eva Mae Edwards (deceased), affectionately known as "granny," for treating me more like a son than just a mere extension of her family. I am truly thankful for her blessings, friendship, love and wisdom— and eternally thankful that she shared this fantastic story with me! I also wish to dedicate this book to my daughter Sabrina, who lost her courageous battle with breast cancer in 2012, and sons Ricky and Keith who preceded her in death.

Contents

Acknowledgments

I am very thankful to be blessed with so many friends and relatives who without their help and patience this book might still be on my computer's hard drive! If not for their positive attitudes, cooperation and encouragement, I might still be stuck in neutral waiting for a push.

Thanks to my lovely wife Sandra for putting up with the clutter and over flowing wastebaskets in our library (my office) and keeping me on the job. Thanks to Judie Wheeler, Jim Wheeler, Willie Mae Martin, Lizzie Asbury, Leon Matthews, Brenda Epperson, Jua Epperson, Tracey Vaughn, Wade Vaughn, George Davis, Frankie Murray, Danielle Parker, Ray Murray,

Terrance Johnson, Sebastian Johnson, Patricia Matlock, and Robert Causey Jr., for their personal testimonials, input, and willingness to share their stories with others. A shout-out to Jean, Sake, Barb, Lee, Ernie, and Ronnie.

A special thanks to Barbara Turner, owner of B Jazz Creations, for her expert help typing, and proofing the many drafts we rejected before submitting the finished manuscript to the publisher. And Terrance L. Johnson, for his invaluable technical assistance and advice, when computer issues beyond my expertise would periodically pop up.

Introduction

Twenty eight years ago I smoked nearly three packs of cigarettes a day: I was a severely addicted chain smoking fool lighting one up after another. Today I am totally free of that debilitating habit, because I learned how to quit smoking COLD TURKEY in ONE day! That's right I quit smoking cigarettes COLD TURKEY in just ONE day — and YOU can too! So don't be dissuaded by the COLD TURKEY reference: It's way overblown! The so-called ill effects associated with quitting smoking COLD TURKEY— are usually overly emphasized and extremely exaggerated — as you will soon discover once you've made the commitment to go that route!

I wrote this book because so many people asked me to write it. Over the years I've shared granny's story with hundreds of people who successfully kicked the habit COLD TURKEY like I did. They followed the instructions I received from granny <u>to the letter</u>. They in turn relayed the exact information to their friends and relatives who had the same success! You will read several of their testimonials interlaced within various tenets throughout this book. The only prerequisite for you to quit smoking COLD TURKEY in ONE day — and never smoke again — is your commitment to do it! It's entirely up to you.

Consider this: you're at home watching television, and the telephone has not rung all day long, and you haven't attempted to use it either. There was no one on your agenda that you had an urge to phone. Then something happens to disrupt your service; why do you all of a sudden think of fifty different people you have to call? The water main breaks, you want to take a shower; the gas is cut off, then you want to make a pizza. The lights go off, and now you want to read a book! What causes this anxiety? The short answer is deprivation: you want it, because you can't have it! Your subconscious mind is messing with you!

To quit smoking cigarettes is also a form of deprivation. You want to light up, but you know you shouldn't — and without your commitment not to light up — you probably will! It's all in your mind but guess what: If you follow the information I share with you in this book, you won't have to deal with any of the aforementioned distractions — because I will tell you HOW to keep that commitment — and quit smoking 'cold turkey' in just ONE day! <u>I will also teach you how not to light up again once you've quit!</u>

Unless you've been living in a cave, under a rock or on the moon, you've probably heard all the pros and cons related to tobacco use in one form or another. So I don't want to bore you with a bunch of regurgitated statistics that I've read someplace in medical journals, pamphlets, magazines and such attempting to validate myself as being an authority on the subject of smoking cessation. I am just the messenger. SO DO NOT SHOOT ME!

However, I would be remiss if I didn't mention the fact that smoking increases your blood pressure, narrows your arteries and promotes plaque buildup which leads to blood clots in your arteries. Smokers also inhale over 4,000 harmful chemicals with each puff, which can destroy lung tissue and increase their risk of getting cancer of the mouth, throat, esophagus, and stomach exponentially. In addition — smoking is said to be responsible for 85% of deaths from (COPD). Now I know why they're called Coffin nails!

I would be equally remiss if I didn't talk about the ills of *secondhand smoke* which was the foremost reason I quit smoking in the first place. Here's the skinny on that subject. The Centers for Disease

Control and Prevention say secondhand and even <u>third</u> hand smoke can cause asthma, respiratory and ear infections, sudden infant death syndrome (SIDS), heart disease and lung cancer. Statistics also reveal that smoking cigarettes kill almost 500,000 people each year — that's over 1,000 people a day — still one in five adults continues to light up! I guess you can lead a horse to water, but you can't make it drink! <u>But, you already know that: Right?</u>

I quit smoking cigarettes over twenty eight years ago (February 12, 1987) but the years of abusing my body had already taken its toll. As a result, I suffer from Chronic Pulmonary Obstruction Disease (COPD) which on occasion requires me to use compressed oxygen to supplement my breathing. Especially when I think I'm still thirty years old and over exert myself attempting to do things I probably couldn't do even when I *was* thirty! In Consideration of my age and disability, I believe I'm in pretty good physical shape.

I still play lots of golf, among a lot of other things that shall remain personal! Ahem: just clearing my throat.

In January of 1987 I was the only person in my household addicted to cigarettes, or I should say nicotine. My wife didn't smoke, my daughter wasn't a smoker, and my son-in - law was also a nonsmoker. My daughter Sabrina was pregnant with her first son, Terrance, and it was rapidly approaching her delivery date. She was due any day now.

I was in the family room watching television when a Public Service Announcement (PSA) aired informing viewers that inhaling secondhand smoke was indeed just as detrimental to the body as actually smoking the real thing! With the voiceover, they displayed a myriad of graphs and images of diseased lungs at various stages of deterioration related to cigarette smoking. The photos were very graphic and left nothing to the imagination! I was like — damn that was some hardcore stuff! Now you know I did NOT say stuff — I said exactly what you thought I said. It blew my mind!

The PSA's are even more graphic today! I assume you've probably seen or heard the many horrific and heartbreaking stories from the perspective of those whose bodies were ravished and mutilated because of their addiction to nicotine.

The testimonial where that once beautiful lady takes off her wig, removes her makeup — and then takes out her dentures to reveal the horrific aftermath caused by smoking cigarettes — should prompt every smoker and tobacco user to head for the nearest trash container!

The first thought that entered my mind when I saw the PSA in 1987 was to kick the habit! I did not want to chance harming the new baby. Although I didn't fully understand what ramifications secondhand smoke could possibly have on the yet to be born baby's tiny organs — I made the conscious decision that grandpa's boy would be coming home to a smoke free environment — and not become an unwilling victim of this deadly ritual! I knew right then and there I was going to quit smoking those cancer sticks!

I also knew this was going to be a humongous challenge, because I had already attempted to quit on several other occasions and failed. The outcome would probably be the same as before. At least that's what I thought. You see, I had successfully completed a certified smoking cessation program — got a certificate — and even quit smoking 'cold turkey' for nearly two weeks! What would be different this time?

In spite of convincing myself I was about to fail once again, something phenomenal happened this time. As fate would dictate, a petite little lady in her eighties revealed to me the tenets that would open the doorway to a new way of life for me, and many others who would quit smoking cigarettes in just ONE day — and never light up again!

I listened intently as granny told me how to eradicate my addiction 'cold turkey' in 24 hours and never start up again. When she finished telling me how this "Lil old white man," as she put it, walked out of this bright light in the middle of the road and blessed her with certain knowledge, I'm like "granny you been drinking?" She warned me not to fall victim to the naysayers and those folks who might wish you ill will, because misery likes company. "Just do what I told you to do Ricky!"

The words she spoke to me that Sunday afternoon, were unbelievable, but hung on my ears like magnets. When I was ready to test the water I followed granny's instructions to a tee — and quit smoking cigarettes 'cold turkey' in just one day! <u>I quit smoking cigarettes 'cold turkey'</u> in one day, and never smoked another! That was over twenty eight years ago, and I have never touched one since! Whoa — I think I touched one — but I didn't smoke it. Look at the person next to you, and say "he touched it, but he didn't smoke it: Hallelujah!"

It's probable that some of you may have quit smoking cigarettes two times or more, but started back again. I've known people who said they quit for as long as FIVE years and started back again! Why did they start back? Why did YOU start back? Read this book and learn how to quit forever! Granny told me how, and when — and I'll tell YOU how and when. <u>Yes: there is a how and when to quit.</u>

People have various reasons why they want to quit smoking. Some of you out there might even relate to my story as to why *you* want to quit smoking. Others might be forced to quit because of employment requirements, health challenges, state or municipal ordinances that ban smoking in bars, casinos, restaurants, sports arenas, and other public venues. Some establishments are even banning the electronic vapor 'e cigarettes'. No smoking signs are even popping up at a number of apartment buildings and condominiums that forbid folks from lighting up in their own homes! Not even in your own bathroom! If you don't quit soon — you'd better stock up on air freshener. Ewe!

Remember when people used to take a lit cigarette to the bathroom as a cover up even if they didn't smoke? You'd be like, "dude, can I borrow a cigarette for my girl — she's got to go!" On the flip side — guys really don't care who's next in line! Enter at your own risk!

I sincerely think you will find this book to be what you've been searching for in your quest to become a nonsmoker. I know you will enjoy reading it with its wealth of information, and logic. When you have finished reading this book in its entirety, and have put the information I've shared with you to the test, I'm certain you too will be able to say *"I quit 'cold turkey' — and I did it in one day!" And from now on when you go — just light a match!* I'm just saying.

First Tenet

————•«(•)»•————

BE HONEST WITH YOURSELF

My quest to be free from tobacco and nicotine began over thirty years ago when I was employed at one of the so called Big Three automobile factories in Detroit Michigan. My plant was located on Piquette Street in midtown near West Grand Boulevard, where the General Motors headquarters was located during that era.

I was required to be on the job and ready to work at 6:30 a.m. Therefore, my day would begin around 5:00 a.m. Monday through Friday, rain or shine, sleet or snow it was the same old routine. That is, unless I volunteered to work overtime — then I had to get started a little earlier! Now don't get me wrong I am not complaining about the job, or the hard labor, because I got paid good money and benefits for the privilege!

What irks me though are people who have never set one foot on the plant floor and claim to be experts on the subject of how we auto workers are over-paid for doing menial labor — which is far from the truth! We worked our butts off in that factory! It was more than just turning nuts and bolts on the assembly line. I can't begin to count the number of new hires who quit within one week, because they couldn't cut the mustard. But that's another story for another time: Let's get back to how I successfully quit smoking nearly 3 packs of cigarettes a day in just twenty four hours!

During the summer months when the temperature inside the factory would occasionally raise above one hundred degrees Fahrenheit, a few of us would congregate on the roof during our coffee breaks to smoke a few butts and try to cool off a little. To tell you the truth though, most of the time we just got hotter and didn't care about the heat, because we still had to get that quick smoke in before the whistle blew! Ugh!

It was especially tough when they banned smoking on the assembly line, because the only time we got the chance to grab a cigarette was during lunch, bathroom breaks, or other contractual breaks that we were entitled to. The nonsmokers applauded the decision. They didn't sympathize with us the least bit.

They didn't know how it was to smell like crap most of the time, or how your nicotine breath and stained teeth reflected the real you! They didn't realize that your spouse or significant other loved the taste of your polluted lips when the two of you kissed! Didn't they know your sweetheart really looked forward to another sleepless night because that hack, hack, hack, sputum producing, phlegm filtered rattle you called a slight cigarette cough kept them awake most of the night? How dare they applaud — we had rights too! Stupidity, knows no boundaries. Hey Forrrrrrrrest! You know what his mama said; don't you?

Needless to say, the smoking ban was short lived once all the smokers began to take three to four bathroom breaks in an hour and production began to suffer as a result. It didn't take management long to figure out what was going on before they were forced to cancel the smoking ban, however ill advised that decision proved to be! *"Smoke, smoke, smoke that cigarette: Smoke, smoke, smoke yourself to death!"*

Isn't it amazing what concerted effort can accomplish when everyone's on the same page? Us smokers, who were in the minority, protested for the right to jeopardize the health and welfare of the nonsmoking majority, and prevailed! Go figure — we won the right to commit suicide and didn't even know it! Be wary of what you ask for. Concerted effort.............?

Speaking of concerted effort, look what the tobacco industry moguls accomplished in just a short period of time. They took a supposedly harmless plant and turned it into a trillion dollar cash cow! And those of us who were foolish enough to suckle on its teat are now attempting to wean ourselves from that nipple because of the inevitable outcome if we continue to light up: i.e. cancer, diabetes, stroke, emphysema, heart failure, obesity, COPD, and even death!

NOBODY KNEW THE RISK'S ASSOCIATED WITH SMOKING. I take that back: THE GENERAL PUBLIC PROBABLY DIDN'T KNOW THE RISK'S ASSOCIATED WITH CIGARETTE SMOKING. BUT I'LL WAGER THE TOBACCO INDUSTRY KNEW THE RISK'S. I guarantee it! "Can I say that without buying a suit?" "*Smoke, smoke, smoke that cigarette: Smoke, smoke, smoke yourself to death!*"

I took my first puff at the age of thirteen. Yep, eighth grade. What about you? Were we stupid or what! Don't you wish you could take it back? I know I do! What prompts a thirteen year old eighth grader to light up in the first place? Some people might say it was peer pressure — but in my case I believe my decision to smoke was based purely on the environment and the culture during that era more than peer pressure. Teenagers in the fifties and sixties associated smoking cigarettes with being hip or cool, because everywhere you looked you saw tobacco use in one form or another.

Nearly everyone you might encounter in your daily activities had a cigarette, cigar, or pipe clamped between his or her lips, or a chaw of tobacco between his cheek and gums. Movie stars, athletes, politicians, Judges, policemen, lawyers, teachers, doctors, preachers, young men, old men, young ladies, old ladies, rich people, poor people, factory workers, white collar workers, undertakers — and of course also included in that mix was yours truly! If you don't believe me, watch a few of the old retro movies on cable television. You'll soon get the picture. You do have cable, right?

People will often ask. "How did you start smoking at such an early age? Where were your parents? How'd you get away with it?" To tell you the truth, not that I've been lying — my mom didn't smoke but it was fairly easy to swipe a couple of butts from my dad's pack which was usually setting somewhere in plain sight. He never attempted to hide them from anyone. After all — they weren't illegal!

Other than sharing smokes with your friends it was pretty obvious our parents were some of our principal enablers, however unaware they were of that fact. Heck, on occasion your folks or even your adult neighbors would send you to the store to purchase cigarettes for them! Nobody asked for ID to verify if you were old enough to buy cigarettes. Vending machines couldn't check your age. Who needed to ask anyway? They already knew you were under-age!

Several storekeepers would even fill beer and wine orders for us kids. You'd go in, give the clerk the note from your folks and they would fill the order. "Let me see, eggs.... bread.... milk.... cheese...wine.... 2 packs of *Old Gold.*" So, do you see how easy it was to buy cigarettes back in the day? I am sooooo glad I quit smoking when I did — besides being a health hazard — cigarettes today are so high you have to buy'em one at a time! Tap your neighbor on the left and say "Where can I buy a loosey?"

I can remember the first time my parents got hip to my cigarette habit. At least I thought it was the first time they had gotten hip to me. I say that, because my sage knowledge today tells me otherwise. How do you hide the smell? You can't! Deodorants, chewing gum, mouthwash, or anything else will mask the odor of tobacco! A nonsmoker can detect the odor of a smoker in his or her sleep. Do you still feel hip...?

You cannot fool a nonsmoker no matter how hard you may try. Some folks might even patronize you by pretending to believe it when you tell them you've quit smoking. They want to spare you the embarrassment of being made a liar, but they do know.

My mom was probably already on to me long before I made my daring move, she being the only nonsmoker in the family. My dad was probably hip to me too — despite his smelling like an ashtray most of the time. Ugh — and my mama had to kiss those nicotine tasting lips — yuck! Did I say that out loud?

So, here we were on our way to Los Angeles, California via automobile. My dad was a Baptist Minister and attended the National Baptist Convention every year. Each year we would pack up and travel to the city hosting the convention. We would travel by automobile, which wasn't too bad, because dad always owned a luxury vehicle with lots of leg room inside. Hold up now, I didn't say it was a brand new luxury vehicle, but it was brand new to us!

I can remember whenever we got a new used car (oxymoron) we would visit friends and relatives all over town just to show off our new used car! Everybody would get to ride around the block in the new car. Most everyone in the neighborhood did the same thing when they upgraded cars. My folks probably should have just called it a "different" used car — because it sure wasn't new! They should have called their friends and said "we just got a different used car today, a 1949 Buick, different color too! Y'all want to see it?" "HELLOOOOO — it's 1957!"

My dad was partial to Cadillac and Buick, both of which had large rear seats that allowed me to stretch out as if I was home in my own bed. So I was pretty comfortable. Plus, on really long trips like this, they would drive until dusk then get us a motel room for the night. That's when the trip seemed almost like a real vacation, and not just something I was a party to by default simply because they didn't trust me to stay at home with my older siblings! I was a baaaaaaad boy! Can you tell?

Occasionally when my parents couldn't get a room in the south, we would drive straight through to our destination. Even with the plush seats, those stretches of 1500 miles one way would still kill you. No motel, hotel, Holiday Inn — the routine was to stop, stretch, pee, and gas up! In addition to *my* pee break behind the gas station, I would sneak in a puff or two, maybe three. Now y'all know I'm black — don't cha? What tipped you off....? Turn to your neighbor and say, "No rooooom at the Inn— he MUST be black!"

We were somewhere near Utah and had traveled over a hundred miles since our last pit stop and

I was having a nicotine fit! You see, I never got the opportunity to catch a smoke at the last pit stop, because I couldn't shake my dad! Everywhere I turned he was there! Now I'm craving a smoke real bad, and in agony from smelling his smoke for a hundred miles or so, praying for the gas gauge to get low so we'd have to gas up again! But, for some reason that damned gas gauge seemed to stand still! <u>That's when I decided to throw caution to the wind and make my move!</u> Dum... ta... dum... dummm............! Tap your neighbor once again and say, "He's about to get his ass whipped!"

When I just couldn't take it anymore I pulled out my smoke's, lit up, and took a drag so deep it damned near choked me to death! My dad glanced at me through the rear-view mirror. I was trying not to make eye contact. He asked me "When did you start smoking?" I told him the truth. He warned me he wouldn't be supporting my habit if I continued to smoke, but considering the fact that I was sixteen years old, the choice was mine to make. Believe it or not that was the extent of our conversation concerning my smoking. He didn't even repeat that old cliché about cigarette smoking stunting your growth, or any of the other bullshit your parents would say to you to discourage you from doing something they didn't agree with. California here we come!

On the other hand, my mom just stared at me and shook her head in disgust. My dad was true to his word though. There were many days when I would resort to smoking his stale ashtray butts because I couldn't afford to buy a pack of my own! Which was no big deal to me, I'd been smoking them anyway for the past three years! *Smoke, smoke, smoke that cigarette: Smoke, smoke, smoke yourself to death!"*

Have you ever lied to a nonsmoker about having successfully quit smoking and thought you had actually fooled them? Don't you feel embarrassed today knowing you didn't fool anyone but yourself? I know I did at one time: walking around smelling like an ashtray, talking about I had quit smoking...........! YOU DID IT TOO!

As I indicated earlier — you cannot fool a nonsmoker! So if you really want to stop smoking <u>the number one tenet is to be honest with yourself!</u> I say this from firsthand experience, because I lied to myself about my desire to quit smoking. I even made several attempts to quit, but without success. I wasn't successful until I was honest about wanting to quit!

I wasn't successful because there was always someone else urging me to quit, and not myself! I was trying to quit for them, and not me! I was attempting to quit smoking hoping to please other people, but deep inside I knew I really wasn't up to the challenge. I was not ready to commit! I would always find a reason not to quit. So in order to be successful *<u>you must be totally honest with yourself.</u>* You have to be up to the challenge to commit when YOU decide to quit! You are the decider: Did I just say that?

△ △ △ △

I can remember when my wife Sandy and I planned a romantic weekend one summer, which was to include a dinner cruise, and a night of dancing and romancing. All day long we talked about how much fun we were about to have later that evening. We even purchased our tickets weeks in advance to assure ourselves a choice table on the boat.

We were running a little late per usual when we left home, as a result we would barely have time to park the car and hightail it to the dock. Wait a minute! I patted my jacket pocket and didn't feel that familiar rectangular soft pack of cigarettes pressing against my chest. I checked the glove box, nothing! My heart began to pound rapidly and I broke out in a cold sweat! Hit me now! Get on up! Get on up! I glanced at my watch — they will stop boarding in twenty minutes, but I have got to get some S- M- O- K- E- S!

I knew they didn't sell cigarettes aboard the boat, so I had to stop along the way to buy a pack. I spied a party store, slammed on my brakes, left the motor running, leapt from the car and ran in to get my nicotine fix! As stupid as it was, I told my wife weeks ago that I had given up the habit— and now I'm about to get busted! Turn to the person on your right, and say, "Uh oh, the smoke's about to hit the fan!"

When we finally arrived downtown we parked the car and made it to the pier just in time to see the boat drifting away from the dock. Needless to say the honeymoon was over that night. Plus — to add insult to injury — she knew I hadn't quit anyway! Smelling like a damn ashtray! *Smoke, smoke, smoke that cigarette: Smoke, smoke, smoke yourself to death!"*

Second Tenet

---◦((◦))◦---

ARE YOU REALLY
READY TO QUIT?

In your quest to give up smoking did you ever try using the nicotine patch, nicotine gum or the electronic cigarette? Have you undergone hypnosis, or an acupuncture procedure? Have you tried any other method of smoking cessation? If so, why did you fail to quit? You don't have the slightest clue, do you? Well, I'll let you in on a secret my friend. *You failed, because you didn't want to quit! It's just that simple!* "What you talking 'bout Willis?"

I'm talking about what most smoking cessation products have in common, and they spell it out in their literature. Here's what they say: They tell you their products will help <u>reduce your nicotine craving while you attempt to quit smoking.</u> Even the so-called e-cigarettes (electronic vapor cigarettes) make the same disclaimer. <u>They don't claim to be a cure for your nicotine habit. They claim you should be able to quit smoking in about 12 weeks without severe cravings!</u>

Some smokers believe e-cigarettes can take the place of quitting 'cold turkey' because they have the option of choosing a placebo cartridge, or still get their nicotine fix through a nicotine cartridge if they so choose. They can even fire up where smoking is prohibited, because e-cigarettes are smokeless, and odorless. Sounds good, huh? Epic fail! Is nicotine still present in the vapor that's expelled from the cartridge, or does it just mysteriously disappear? The jury is still out on that one, but the fat lady is warming up her vocal cords: ahem! Tap somebody on the shoulder and say "she's tuning up!"

NEWSFLASH! *You have to want to quit smoking if you are to be successful!* Let me repeat that phrase. *You have to want to quit smoking if you are to be successful!* So if you really want to quit smoking you have to be honest with yourself, or you are doomed to failure before you even begin.

The good news is, I know the secret that will enhance your chances of being successful, and I am going to share it with you in this book. That's right; everything you need to know is contained within these pages! There's absolutely nothing else to purchase. No gum, no patches, no shots, no hypnotherapy, no acupuncture no electronic cigarettes, nothing else — because it's all here!

Plus, you won't have to experience any of the unpleasant side effects that may be associated with the aforementioned, which might include nausea, vomiting, headaches, dizziness, spasms, blurred vision, double vision, triple vision, nosebleeds, diarrhea, earaches, toothaches, stained fingernails, erectile dysfunction, under arm odor, hair loss, (men) facial hair growth, (women) sleep apnea, cramps, bloating, insomnia, hearing loss, constipation, flatulence, bad breath, and impotence. The entire list of possible side effects could not be printed at this time because of its volume. Sorry y'all......but take my word, they aren't good!

In the first tenet I strongly emphasized the need to be honest with yourself, and believe me, that advice alone is the key that will unlock the door to your success! I point this out, because if you try to fool yourself into believing you can be weaned off cigarettes by cutting back — EPIC FAIL! If you think you can chew nicotine gum or use an electronic cigarette regimen to break your addiction — EPIC FAIL! If you think someone can hypnotize you into quitting your smoking habit permanently — EPIC FAIL! If you rationalize that a little nicotine will ease your craving for cigarettes until you quit — EPIC FAIL!

So save yourself some money by not being duped into thinking you have to spend hundreds, or maybe even thousands of dollars on pills, patches, chewing gum, hypnosis, acupuncture, and all sorts of other gimmicks that promise to make it easier for you to break your habit — because I don't believe they will!

None of the above will work for any length of time, because as I said before, you have already set yourself up for failure long before even getting started. Why? Because you've already admitted to yourself that you can't quit on your own without utilizing the gimmicks I mentioned above. You want to take the easy way out, but in essence what you've done is to inform your subconscious mind you want to fail. Because there is no easy way out! <u>You're going to have to suck it up and quit 'cold turkey' just like those of us who have successfully quit smoking and have not started back</u>

<u>again. You have to stop blowing smoke and JUST QUIT!</u> "You heard me..........?"

Here's the deal. You cannot substitute one form of nicotine delivery for another and somehow think you're suddenly going to become an ex-smoker! What happens when you stop chewing the gum, smoking the e-cigarette, or wearing the patch that's supplying the nicotine to your system? I'll tell you what's going to happen. One of the following: You're going to quit 'cold turkey' — start smoking once again — or continue to use the so called aid and remain addicted! <u>There can be no other plausible outcome.</u>

Using a nicotine patch or e-cigarette hoping to wean one's self off cigarettes is akin to a heroin addict switching to methadone while attempting to break his addiction to heroin. In which case, the synthetic drug is just as detrimental to his success of quitting as the real thing! The fact remains he's merely substituting one drug addiction for another. It's a no win situation.

Be it drugs, alcohol, or tobacco the end result will be the same. You cannot tell your subconscious mind that you only wish to *cut down* a little bit: Either you want to quit, or you don't. There is no in between. Your subconscious mind will only obey what you have programmed it to do. As a result you will continue to be a part time drug addict, alcoholic, or as in your case, a part time smoker!

I'll wager you know, or have known a few people who fit the above profile. I know I do. Here's some food for thought. If you don't believe you are ready to make the commitment to quit smoking at this time — close this book and put it on the shelf until you are really ready to fully commit. Otherwise you're just setting yourself up to fail once again. The bottom line is this, when you administer that so called "final" dose of nicotine, however miniscule it may be, the end result will still be the same, 'COLD TURKEY' whether it's in the form of gum, patch, e-cigarette, or any other method of delivery. <u>And I believe that's a fact that</u> <u>cannot be disputed!</u>

Δ Δ Δ Δ

My wife's cousin, a retired registered nurse, was a pack a day smoker before kicking the habit. She said she felt like a hypocrite knowing the dangers associated with cigarette smoking, because of her profession, but nevertheless made the choice to continue smoking. She would light up the first thing in the morning and by the time she arrived at the hospital where she worked — she would have smoked two or three cigarettes. Cousin Bill (short for Willie Mae) would light up during coffee breaks and at lunch, or any other situation that afforded her the opportunity to light up.

When I told her the story I'm about to share with you later on, Bill flat out told me she was not ready to quit, because she truly enjoyed smoking cigarettes! She also indicated cigarette smoking helped her to cope with the stressful working conditions associated with her occupation. Bill said when the time comes for her to quit smoking she would know it and would deal with it then, but until then, she would continue to enjoy her habit.

A couple of years later I saw Bill at a family reunion in New York, and she had kicked the habit! I asked her how did she overcome the desire to keep smoking, and what she said was something I never suspected. She told me she knew it was time for her to quit after witnessing a terminally ill patient who had smoked cigarettes for over forty years or more lose his battle with lung cancer. She told me after watching that patient suffer the way he did before he died, convinced her enough was enough! At that she said she remembered what I had shared with her back in Detroit and decided to give it a try.

Although she was able to quit smoking overnight, Bill never-the-less kept an unopened pack of cigarettes in her purse for over two months! She concluded, just knowing she could always reach into her pocket for a smoke if she really needed one was reassuring. That unopened pack of cigarettes became a security blanket of sorts to help her get through the day. When she was truly convinced that she was no longer a slave to nicotine — she tossed the pack of cigarettes into the trash and the rest was history.

Here is the consummate example of what I have been saying all along. In this case my wife's cousin knew she wasn't really ready to quit smoking, so she didn't set herself up for failure by even trying. <u>Bill waited until the time came when she knew</u> <u>without a doubt that she was ready to quit.</u> Even then she carried a pack of cigarettes in her purse or on her person for over two months as a stress reliever: *"Smoke, smoke, smoke that cigarette: Smoke, smoke, smoke yourself to death!"*

Third Tenet

————— ⮞«❖»⮜ —————

YOU MUST REPROGRAM YOUR SUBCONSCIOUS MIND

I have been fortunate enough to be able to play a little golf at least two or three rounds a week weather permitting. When I am at my best I can visualize the outcome of the shot that I want to hit in my mind's eye before I address the ball. I can mentally see the flight of the ball in the air, watch it land softly on the putting green and roll close to the hole. Then I am able to replay that same visualization when I actually strike the ball, and achieve a like result quite often.

How can this be true you ask? Because, I gave my subconscious mind the blue print for a good shot, and it could only recreate what it saw! The same thing holds true if I start to doubt myself, and my ability to hit good shots. In this case, I will have programmed my mind to hit a bad shot. And as before, my subconscious mind will obey! Once again — garbage in, garbage out! By the way, I do have a hole in one and numerous two shot eagles! They say holes in one come easy after you get your first. Don't believe it! I've come close a few times after my first one, but no cigar. Did I just say cigar....? Hated them!

When I was in the early stages of writing this book I came across an article in my local newspaper about a drug and alcohol residential rehabilitation treatment facility that was having a hard time financially, because of lack of funding and various other problems. In spite of the situation, the facility was still doing its best to help the residents with their addictions.

The reporter who wrote the story had interviewed two of the residents concerning their addictions, and their stories really caught my eye, because both of them hit the nail on the head as it related to addiction, dependency, and the mind.

One of the men was addicted to drugs and the other man was hooked on booze. The two had been severely addicted in excess of twenty years, and each had been in rehabilitation facilities many times. After their release both men had managed to stay clean a week or two here, and a month or so there — but neither man was able to sustain sobriety for any prolonged period of time. They kept falling off the wagon! Time and time again both men tried to divest themselves of their addictions, but time after time each of them failed to stay sober.

Why did they fail to maintain sobriety when released back into society after successfully completing the program? The CEO of the facility put it this way. "The

<u>people here generally have already been in treatment elsewhere, and relapsed: Because addiction is a disease that is characterized by relapse</u>s. Let's take a look at the common characteristics instrumental in keeping each man from achieving lasting sobriety.

The first man was a teacher who got hooked on crack cocaine. He robbed banks to finance his habit and eventually ended up doing six years in a state prison. He said he could get the crack out of his system, *but not out of his mind*! Three weeks after his release he was back in crack's merciless grip. All it took was three weeks on the street for him to <u>relapse!</u>

Then there's the other man, the alcoholic. When he didn't drink he could make a decent living in his given line of work, but that wasn't very often in a life which took him through several of the best regarded residential treatment programs for alcoholics in the state. Nothing took except booze. *"I couldn't change my frame of thinking. I always ended up the same."* He said.

Both of these men came to the same conclusion about their addictions. *They discovered they could live with the <u>physiological</u> aspect of their addiction — but could not overcome the <u>psychological</u> aspect of their addiction! This is true in most cases, which reinforces my assertion that in order to be truly free from your addiction to cigarettes you must reprogram your thoughts! <u>You must reprogram your way of thinking! You must want to quit! You must be honest with yourself! Most of all, you must unlock your mind and reprogram it for success!</u>*

How does one reprogram one's mind you ask? Consider the following: How many times have you attempted to quit smoking, but could not stop thinking about cigarettes until you finally lit up again? You didn't relapse and light up again because your body all of a sudden demanded nicotine. After two or three days, your system will probably be devoid of nicotine anyway. <u>You relapsed, because you could not</u>

overcome your mental craving to continue smoking! You relapsed, because *you failed to reprogram your subconscious mind!*

Consequently, your subconscious mind kept nagging you to smoke until you finally lit up again! It knew your body was accustomed to the benefits derived from the physiological aspect of your addiction, i.e. the aroma, the touch, the taste, and the ritual of literally blowing smoke! Your subconscious mind knew your many weaknesses and preyed upon them causing you to relapse!

Every addiction has a psychological aspect as well as a physiological aspect associated with such addiction. Therefore, if you divest yourself from one aspect of said addiction — you must also free yourself from the other. Why did the drug addict and the alcoholic relapse time after time? Because they couldn't overcome the mental aspect of their addiction!

Cigarette smoking and nicotine addiction is no different. When you quit smoking <u>physically</u> — you must also quit smoking <u>mentally</u> as well! You must reprogram your subconscious mind to forget about smoking cigarettes! Otherwise — you're going to continue to smoke cigarettes while attempting to satisfy your <u>physical</u> graving for nicotine — when in fact the real culprit holding you hostage is your <u>mental</u> craving for nicotine! Your ability to come to grips with, and deal with the psychological and the physiological aspect of the condition people refer to as the <u>disease</u>, has been compromised by your inability to discern the difference between the two!

Have you on occasion listened to a song, a jingle, or a catchy tune on the radio or television only to discover later you couldn't get it out of your mind? I believe the scientific definition for this phenomenon is called an "earworm." No matter what you did to expunge that tune from your thoughts it kept popping up all day long, didn't it? Do you remember what you did to finally get it out of your mind? Probably not — but I'll tell you what you did. You made a <u>conscious</u> effort to think about something other than that jingle. *<u>You reprogrammed your subconscious mind — and you didn't even know it!</u>*

Now I don't profess to be an authority on the subject of psychodynamics, but I do know it works! I practice it every day. Behavioral Science, Psycho Cybernetics, Positive Mental Attitude, Self- Talk, Self-Hypnosis, Subliminal Learning, Cognitive Behavioral Therapy, no matter what you label the concept they all have the same basic meaning, which consists of the following: A method by which we can program our subconscious mind to influence our mental thought process to facilitate a desired outcome. It is a way by which we can change our limited belief system by <u>deprogramming and reprogramming our minds!</u>

Simply put — Psychodynamics is the psychology of what causes us to believe what we believe. A man is what he believes himself to be — if he is not, he soon will become what he believes himself to be! Therefore if you truly believe what I am about to reveal to you and you really want to quit smoking you will be successful! If you see yourself as a nonsmoker you soon will become a nonsmoker. What one can conceive one can achieve! That's not just a cliché — it happens to be true!

△ △ △ △

I had a very dear friend who was a two pack a day smoker, and a little overweight. He was also a business colleague in my line of work, which was organized labor. I believe it was sometime during the spring of 1997 when we both attended a conference in Washington DC and we were lodging at a hotel on Connecticut Avenue near the infamous "Watergate Office Complex."

I remember bumping into Leon in our hotel lobby one morning as I was leaving for my morning walk in the park. He asked me where I was off to, so I told him that I was about to take a walk in the park behind the hotel. He asked me if he could join me since he was just about to go out for a walk himself. I said I'd be delighted to have him come along. Given the fact that we hadn't seen one another for quite a while this would afford us a good opportunity to catch up on old times.

Mind you, we had to go down a steep hill that was nearly two blocks long to get to the park, and we had to traverse the same route to get back to the hotel. When we completed our jaunt in the park we started back to our hotel. When we approached the stretch that included the steep hill, Leon's breathing became labored, and he motioned for me to slow down a little. Little did he know, I was about to stop anyway! Although I hadn't touched a cigarette in over ten years, the thirty plus years of smoking over two packs a day had already taken its toll! My lungs were shot: Emphysema!

I believe we stopped to rest several times before we were halfway up that hill! We even joked about hailing one of the several taxicabs that had passed us on our laborious trek up what seemed like Mt. Everest to the two of us! In between his huffing and puffing, Leon lamented about his inability to kick his cigarette addiction, and his desire to get in better shape. I even pretended to be Redd Foxx the comedian feigning a heart attack: "Elizabeth honey, I'm coming home to join you. I'll be with a little short fat dude in a green jogging suit, who got hit by a bus, while trying to flag down a taxi."

It was during one of these several rest stops that I told him what was revealed to me on the subject — knowing it would help him with his quest to quit smoking. He thanked me and told me he had attempted to kick the habit many times before to no avail, and at this point in his life he was willing to try just about anything! He said he had nothing to lose and everything to gain! We both laughed, and continued to huff and puff up that steep assed hill. *"Smoke, smoke, smoke that cigarette: Smoke, smoke, smoke yourself to death!"*

Several years had passed before I saw my friend Leon again, and as always, we were very delighted to see one another. I was amazed at his physical condition! He appeared to have shed a few pounds, and he looked as if he were ten years younger. As fate would dictate, I was standing in for my boss at this meeting, and Leon was hosting the meeting in his boss' stead. Ironically, the key note speaker couldn't make it to the hall in time due to a family emergency, so I got railroaded into becoming the keynote speaker! Not to worry though, because I always kept a generic speech in my briefcase at all times just for occasions such as this.

When he introduced me as the keynote speaker, Leon shared some of what I had told him during our walk in Washington with the audience. I was taken aback when he told them I was responsible for changing his life! I discovered he had taken what I had revealed to him on that steep hill in Washington DC, applied it — and had not smoked a cigarette since! You can't imagine what an impact that statement had on me. I was flabbergasted!

During our visit after the meeting, Leon told me he had shared the story I told him in D.C. with several of his friends who were also really ready to quit smoking. They had also successfully kicked the habit! He reinforced what I already knew! _To be successful, you must want to quit! If you do, you will!_

If it's your desire to stop smoking with hopes of insuring yourself a chance at a longer, healthier life, ask yourself — are you really ready to quit? Are you really ready to go the distance without relying on the crutches that I alluded to in the first paragraph of this tenet? Are you really ready to reprogram your subconscious mind for success and divest yourself of all the things waiting to doom you to failure even before you get started? If so, just like my friend Leon, and many others who have successfully quit smoking, you will be well on your way to enjoying a nicotine free, smoke free, healthier existence also!

Fourth Tenet

REPROGRAMING
YOUR SUBCONSCIOUS MIND

How does one deprogram and reprogram one's mind? I know you're anxiously awaiting that revelation, so let me begin by assuring you that the process of deprogramming, and reprogramming ones subconscious mind is relatively simple. The first component is relaxation. You must be able to free your mind and body of pent up stress, frustration, and all other outside distractions in order to be in a total relaxed state of mind.

Some folks might consider what I am about to share with you a form of self - hypnosis, but I can assure you it's only one of several methods used to transform your mind and body into a relaxed state of being. So regardless the terminology it all boils down to whether or not you believe in the process. If you believe in the process you will be successful, and if you don't believe in the process you will fail. It's just that simple — so think positive!

In the second tenet I talked about an addiction having two components within its makeup. First there's the <u>physiological</u> aspect of the dependency, and then there's the <u>psychological</u> aspect of the dependency. Consequently, when you divest yourself from one aspect of the dependency — you must divest yourself of the other aspect of the dependency as well, or you will not be successful.

Do you remember when I talked about the drug addict and the alcoholic, and how they could free themselves from the physical aspect of their addictions, but neither could overcome the mental aspect of his addiction? They both relapsed time after time again, didn't they? <u>Cigarette smoking and nicotine addiction is no different</u>. When you <u>physically</u> quit smoking cigarettes — you must also quit smoking cigarettes <u>mentally</u> as well. You must deprogram — then reprogram your subconscious mind!

The first component in the process is to relieve oneself of all stress! You must be in a totally relaxed state — mind and body. It is imperative that you free your mind of all stress related minutiae that may be imbedded in your subconscious as it will impede the visualization process you are about to experience.

I want you to find a nice quiet place where you will be able to relax without interruption for at least fifteen to twenty minutes. Pop an easy listening instrumental into your CD player, or click on your IPod, then take the most comfortable position available for relaxation, be it your favorite chair, sofa, bed, or even the floor.

If unable to devote fifteen minutes or more to this exercise for any reason, it's acceptable to limit the breathing component of the exercise to 2 or 3 minutes, and the visualization component to 5 or 10 minutes if necessary. You will still attain satisfactory benefits when using these suggested modifications.

Deep breathing exercises have been one of various proven methods used to help relieve stress in folks active in a myriad of professions, from athletes, dancers, orators, and musicians; to stockbrokers, school teachers, and airline pilots to name a few. A proven stress reliever I use is a deep breathing exercise I learned from granny that she coined "smell the cake and blow out the candle." Believe it or not, I discovered that many yoga instructors teach similar breathing technique's in their sessions. How did granny know? Beats me........?

Whenever you become overwhelmed with the desire to smoke and inundated with stress: gather yourself — close your eyes and inhale through your nose while mentally counting up to 4 — hold for 4 counts then exhale (as though blowing out candles on a cake) as you mentally count up to 8. Your diaphragm should expand when you inhale and contract as you exhale. Repeat at least five times then gradually resume your normal breathing pattern. As you inhale and exhale, peace and tranquility will engulf your very being as the stress seeps from your extremities (hands, feet, arms, legs, etc.) <u>The urge to light up will</u> <u>even go away after a few minutes.</u> Trust me — it works!

Once you have resumed your normal breathing pattern — I want you to relax, and replay in your mind the most enjoyable stress free and relaxing situation that you can conjure up (real or fantasy). I want you to re-live such experience and immerse yourself into that scenario as if it were truly happening. Make it in the now! Daydream — we do it all the time!

If your place of serenity was an ocean front beach in the tropics, visualize yourself in that beautiful island paradise at sunset on a warm sandy beach. Feel the warm breeze as it caresses your face, smell the freshness of nature entering your nostrils while your gaze catches the burnt orange highlights of the setting sun. Listen to the sound of the white tipped waves lapping the shoreline in rhythmic synchronization, ebbing and flowing to the beat of mother-nature. Take yourself to that place and be a part of your visualization. Immerse yourself into that scenario. Can you see the palm trees swaying in the distance? Can you smell the fresh ocean breeze? Hear the sounds, feel the sand beneath your feet — breathe in the aromas. Be in the moment! Relax. Relax. Relax.

When you have utilized this technique a few times it will become easier and easier to relax and visualize yourself in any situation or destination you may choose. <u>It's all in your mind! Relax and enjoy the serenity</u>

Fifth Tenet

——•«◉»•——

STOP MAKING EXCUSES

How many times have you told yourself you would quit smoking if you could only figure out how not to gain weight? You concluded this, because some people who quit smoking for any length of time said they gained a considerable amount of weight, and *you* don't want to get fat. Am I correct? What about this one? "I would stop smoking if I could still drink my morning coffee, because I *know* I would still crave my morning caffeine and I'm accustomed to smoking two or three cigarettes with my coffee. Here's another one. "I've got to smoke whenever I have a drink — and I just love having an occasional cocktail." This one is the best of all. "I can quit whenever I choose — it's just that I'm not ready to quit right now." *"Smoke, smoke, smoke that cigarette: Smoke, smoke, smoke yourself to death!"*

PEOPLE...you cannot continue to make excuses, if you really want to quit smoking! It would be reasonable to rationalize that you would not be reading this book if you weren't the least bit curious of its contents and perhaps its relevance to your plight. If this is the case, I am certain you will be enlightened and your curiosity sated as you continue reading the ensuing tenets. But first you have to stop making excuses to not quit smoking!

In the first and second tenets, I stressed over and over that you would have to be honest with yourself and must really be ready to quit! And now in this fifth tenet I am suggesting you stop making excuses as to why you can't — or shouldn't quit! Unless you can truly embrace the above advice, commit to it wholeheartedly, and adhere to it — you will continue to search for the easy way out. Success will only continue to elude you, because as I stated in the second tenet — there *is* no easy way out!

You contend that you might gain a little weight if you quit smoking. So what! Unless you're a model, or a movie star, who cares if you've gained a few pounds? I gained a little weight when I quit smoking, but as I began walking a few miles every day, in addition to watching my diet, my weight began to drop accordingly. Above all, I know I'm in pretty decent shape. I also know I am not twenty years old either!

Without a doubt you'll probably gain weight anyway as you age — even if you <u>do</u> continue to smoke with the false belief that smoking will keep you thin. Now, I'm not advocating that aging and weight gain go hand in hand. However, if you don't exercise, or maintain a healthy diet you're still going to gain a pound or two anyway — trust me! But, at least if you quit smoking, even with the chance of gaining a little booty — you'll probably live longer and your food's going to taste a whole lot better! And as for you twenty year old readers — you might even live to be a hundred!

Before we leave the subject of weight gain I want to share something I read in a Fitness Magazine about *stress* and weight gain. According to the American Psychological Association, a whopping 75% of people in the United States feel stressed out, and almost half of us eat unhealthy because of it — 47% of us can't sleep because of it. It makes one in three of us depressed and for 42% of us — it has gotten worse in the last year.

The article went on to say stress doesn't just mess with your head, it also messes with your waistline. When you're faced with a nerve wracking situation, your body increases production of the hormone cortisol, part of what experts call the fight-or-flight response. If the stress inducing situation disappears your body returns to normal.

What if the stress remains? Well, that's the problem. The kind of stress most of us face is the ongoing sort which keeps cortisol levels elevated for days. It's that increased cortisol level, in turn, that appears to encourage the body to store additional abdominal fat.

An expanding belly is just one side effect of a stressed out life. Stress is associated with just about every chronic disease we know. Heart disease, diabetes, depression and some cancers are notable examples. Recent research indicates that stress may also be responsible for encouraging addictive behaviors and other unhealthy habits by disrupting the part of your brain responsible for self control and decision making.

I especially wanted to share that last paragraph with you because I can remember lighting one cigarette after another whenever I felt stressed out. When I quit smoking I substituted food for cigarettes! Based on my own personal experiences, and observations, I've concluded that relieving the stressful situations in your life, along with exercise will greatly benefit you in your quest to quit smoking. So stop making excuses, and get on with it!

You long time smokers can reap additional healthful rewards from quitting now: Your blood pressure and pulse rate can decrease within 24 hours, and your pulmonary and circulatory systems can improve in 2-12 weeks. The risk of coronary heart disease may be half that of a smokers in 1 year—and in 10 years the risk of lung cancer is half that of a smokers. So stop making excuses, and get on with it!

∆ ∆ ∆ ∆

A close friend, whom I've known for over forty years, was in town to attend the funeral services of a mutual acquaintance. After the service I invited him to my home, because he said he was bored at the hotel where he shared a suite with his two brothers who had driven from Ohio with him — plus we hadn't seen one another for a few years, so this would be a good time to catch up on old times.

When I picked him up at his hotel it was raining. It was that light, misty, bone chilling rain you sometimes get in October and November in Michigan. Although it wasn't extremely cold outside it was still a bit uncomfortable with the dampness and all. When I pulled up to the entrance of the hotel, there he was with his shoulders scrunched up puffing on a coffin nail, while at the same time trying to stay warm. When he spotted me he flipped his cigarette butt into the drizzle, hopped in and settled into the warm, leather, seat that enfolded him.

When we arrived at my house I introduced my friend George, to my family before we retreated to my "Man Cave" on the lower level. My man cave used to be our basement, but after we remodeled the space it became the lower level, according to my wife — but I still call it my man cave! Especially — when she's not around!

My home boy and I had a great visit in my wife's new lower level. We must have discussed every topic known to man <u>without incident</u> before I drove him back to his hotel. One of the topic's we discussed that night was the very subject you are reading about today — "How to quit smoking."

The reason I underscored the fact that we encountered no incidents during our visit is a reminder of what could have been — because when this guy gets a drink or two into his system — he will make you rue the day you ever met him!

If the discussion was about cars: he could drive as well as, if not better than Richard Petty! If the subject was boxing: He knew more than the Marquis of Queensbury and Muhammad Ali put together! If it's pool, he could beat Minnesota Fats with one hand tied behind his back! Aviation: The Wright brothers didn't know how wrong they were! And please — don't mention religion! Not only did he know everything about scripture, he would even challenge you to a fistfight, if you disagreed with his position too stringently! But, as I stated above, we had a pleasant visit that night because I felt sorry for his two brothers back at the hotel, and accordingly, I monitored his alcohol consumption.

As the evening wore on, George noticed I hadn't smoked a cigarette all night, so he asked me if I had quit smoking 'cold turkey', or by some other method. He was amused at my answer. I told to him the same thing I'm about to reveal to you later in this book. However, he just could not fathom how something so simple could have such an influence on one's psyche. He flat out told me that he considered me to be a very intelligent man, but what I had told him was absolute bullshit! He was a little bit tipsy by then, but not quite over the edge! I laughed and told him to try it for himself, and see what happens, and left it at that. Maybe we avoided an incident, because I didn't let him drink me out of house and home!

My buddy assured me if he really wanted to, he could quit smoking whenever he chooses, and furthermore, anything I could do he could also do! Case in point: When we were young men living in the projects, we were competing "bootleg barbers" in our neighborhood. He professed to be the best! According to him, he could cut hair better than I, he was more proficient at edge ups than I, and he could definitely style hair better than I. Nevertheless, I would always remind him that it was I who had the most customers. He would argue that I had more clients, because I charged less! To make a long story short, my old friend boasted that whenever he was ready to quit smoking he would, and not a day sooner. And that was that.

A little over a year had elapsed before I saw George again. I was fortunate to be one of two people selected by the folks from our hometown to be honored at their annual banquet for our achievements as business people, unionists, and our contributions to society. George was in attendance along with some of his family members and other friends from Texas and Los Angeles.

During the social hour we all got together and talked about how wonderful everyone looked, and how our family members were getting along. You know, "who got married, who got divorced, grandchildren, how do you manage to keep looking so young, etc.!" Pass me my boots, it's getting deep! Some of us weren't even smoking, but we were all blowing lots of it! Come on, you've done it too!

It was during this conversation that George encouraged me to recapitulate to the group what I shared with him that night at my home relative to quitting smoking in one day. I obliged and told them the same story I had recited to him — word for word.

When I finished telling the story George asked if anyone of them believed what they just heard. One man said he didn't know, but maybe it was worth a try. Another man took a swig of beer, belched, and said, "Who knows?" On the other hand, George informed me that he would give it a shot just to prove I was full of shit! Yep, he was drunk as a skunk by then. *Smoke, smoke, smoke that cigarette: Smoke, smoke, smoke yourself to death!"*

In August of 2009 I traveled to Ohio to attend my baby brother's funeral. My friend George was also in attendance. After the interment ceremony we all returned to the church banquet hall for repast. Following the meal, I ventured outdoors to get a breath of fresh air— it was extremely warm inside. I bumped into George, who was chatting with a couple of our classmates from high school. I asked if they were outside getting in a quick smoke, and to my surprise George spoke up and told me that he had not smoked a cigarette since I shared my story with him at my honorarium banquet three years prior!

He went on to say if he hadn't tried it personally he never would have believed it in a million years! However, he still questioned how something so simple could work! He tried it, and he succeeded— but he still couldn't believe it!

I believe my friend's success qualifies what I discussed in tenets one and two, whereby you have to be honest with yourself and really be ready to quit. In this instant case, George was truly ready to quit smoking so everything else was secondary in comparison to that goal. At this point in time he didn't care, or wasn't concerned how inconceivable the method appeared to be — he was willing to try anything now—<u>because he was really ready to quit smoking!</u> Once he made up his mind to quit, the rest came fairly easy. First he submitted, then he committed!

What about you? Are you fully committed — or are you still making excuses? I'll bet some of you have probably given up trying to quit smoking altogether, because of so many failed attempts to do so in the past. Haven't you? If either question applies to you don't worry, because the solution that will emancipate you from your addiction is right there in your hands! Don't be dismayed because you haven't been as successful as you would have liked in your prior attempts. The reason you and so many others have failed to quit is because you didn't know *how* to quit! This time will be different, because for the first time in your quest, you will have the benefit of knowing when, and how to quit smoking. <u>Yes — there is an optimum time to quit smoking also!</u>

While waiting for Sabrina to finish her weekly medical procedure, I struck up a conversation about smoking cessation with a gentleman who was there waiting for his wife to finish her treatment also. He informed me that he and his wife were smokers, and neither could quit for any length of time before starting back. He indicated that he had quit smoking for two years at one time, but started back up when he was laid off from his job. I asked what caused him to start up again after two years. He told me he couldn't manage the stress of not being able to provide his family with the lifestyle they were accustomed to. I also asked him what influenced him to quit smoking for the two years. He said his grandfather was an instrumental force in that decision.

Apparently his grandfather told him that his body would let him know the right time to quit. He was told there was a certain time of the year when you could quit just about any bad habit you might be strapped with. The man said his grandfather's observation was obviously correct, because one day he just got a funny feeling (his words, not mine) and decided to quit, and he did. COLD TURKEY!

Recently I ran into a friend of mine at the pet supply store where I usually shop for my little Yorkie. He used to work at my old GM plant as a line supervisor when I worked there in the seventies. During our chance meeting he told me he had a stent implanted into his artery due to a partial blockage that caused a heart attack in 2009. I inquired about his cigarette habit, because he was a heavy smoker when I knew him in the factory. He told me he had quit smoking six years before his heart attack! When I asked how did he come to quit— he said, "The only way to go — cold turkey!" I gave him a "high - five", and wished him well!

Do you remember in the Introduction of this book when I said I knew I was going to quit smoking when my grandson was born? Do you remember what else I said? Let me remind you. I said, "I didn't know *how* I was going to quit!" Didn't I? That was the primary reason I had failed so many times! I did not know when, and how to quit! Now I do, and so will you as you continue to read and digest the information I am sharing with you in this book.

Sixth Tenet

PREPARE FOR SUCCESS

In earlier tenets I talked about positive attitudes, and how a positive attitude would be invaluable in your quest to quit smoking. So, if you don't believe you are truly ready to quit smoking cigarettes at this time — be honest — and don't set yourself up for failure. Wait until you are certain that you are really ready to quit before you make the commitment. You will know when that time comes.

I included this tenet, because it will test your resolve to quit smoking. You will soon learn as you continue to read these passages, there is indeed an optimum time to stop smoking cigarettes, and this tenet may aid in your successful transformation. Various cessation programs include similar advice in their talking points, instructions or literature with the belief that such rituals have merit in aiding you in your quest to quit smoking.

Although I do agree that a limited amount of placebo relief may be realized as a temporary fix until your chosen quit day arrives: This tenet is not intended as a prerequisite for you to be successful in your endeavor. As you will soon discover in a later tenet, I continued to smoke right up to my designated quit day!

Let me be clear about this tenet. This tenet is not a requirement for your success, but if you are not 100% committed to the challenge — you will fail! On the other hand, if you believe you are up to the challenge and ready to quit — this tenet might aid in your preparation for a successful transformation. So in that regard, you may want to consider implementing the following as part of your daily routine until your designated quit day:

- Boast about what you are about to do.
- Tell your family, friends, and co-workers that you intend to quit smoking.
- Give them the time and date that you intend to initiate your quest, and then set about doing it!
- Think positive. Get into the right frame of mind. Be confident, be self-assured, and be ready to succeed!
- Write down the reason, or reasons you want to quit. Review daily.
- Write down those occasions, events, or other circumstances that compels you to light up, then work on eliminating them from your daily routine (i.e., alcohol, coffee, tea, stress, spouse, significant other, etc.) **
- Remove the ashtrays from your home, car and workplace. Ask family members and co-workers

to refrain from smoking in your presence if possible. Tell them why. Ask for their help.

- Substitute an alternative oral object in place of a cigarette, should you get the urge to light up. For example, chew a stick of sugarless gum instead of smoking, or pop a piece of sugar free hard candy into your mouth. Nibble on a carrot stick, a stalk of celery — drink a glass of water or juice. Some folks even keep a toothpick in the corner of their mouths most of the time.

- Keep busy. Get a hobby, exercise, take a walk, mow the lawn, go to the gym, etc. Most importantly, do something that reinforces your desire to quit smoking! <u>And don't forget to incorporate the deep breathing exercise I</u> <u>talked about in the fifth tenet, should you get the urge to light up.</u>

- Finally, drink plenty of water, eat plenty of fruits and green vegetables (a good source of antioxidants) exercise, or walk at least three days a week for thirty minutes each day. <u>Be sure to check with your physician before starting any exercise or diet program.</u>

- ** (You can keep your spouse or significant other if you must)

When I earned my smoking cessation certificate in 1979, it was as if they expected the participants to fail, because we were always reminded that failure went hand in hand with success! It was like — don't stop trying to quit — some people have relapsed seven to ten times before they experienced any success! <u>Ten times!</u> It didn't work for me either! I was smoking again in two weeks! Chewing toothpicks gets old after a while!

What happened? How did I manage to fall off the wagon in such a short period of time? <u>I relapsed, because I wasn't taught how not to relapse!</u> I wasn't taught to deprogram and reprogram my subconscious mind! I was not taught about what I call "<u>dual addiction</u>

syndrome" (the mental and physical aspect of the addiction), or how to visualize success! In essence — <u>I was not taught how to quit blowing smoke!</u>

But, guess what? As you continue reading this book, you will have the benefit of not only knowing how to quit, you will also learn when to quit — and do it once and for all! I'm going to tell you how to quit smoking <u>COLD TURKEY</u> in just ONE day! Twenty four hours! I did it over 25 years ago and never had the urge to smoke since! You can do it too! But you have to trust what I tell you wholeheartedly if you are to prevail.

I believe some readers may question why I constantly stress failure to be imminent if the tenets I've shared with you thus far are not taken seriously and followed to the letter. Put it this way — failure is the <u>only</u> option if you don't!

If you've attempted to quit smoking in the past why have you failed to remain a nonsmoker? How many times have you attempted to stop smoking in a given period of time? Was it more than twice — three times or more? Why then, are you still addicted? How many failed attempts will you experience before you finally realize that you're going in circles? If you're not convinced that I'm correct — smell your fingers!

You have probably heard the definition of insanity to be "repeating the same mistake over and over but expecting a different result! That's exactly what people think who believe it takes numerous failures before success finds you. That is just not true! You don't have to try to quit smoking five, six or more times to be a nonsmoker! But, you can't get it done until you change your paradigm and do something different when what you are doing is not working! It only makes sense.

If you follow and adhere to the tenets I have shared with you up to this point, and until you've completed this book — you will become a nonsmoker overnight! You just have to man or lady up and get on with it! You can do it: It's all in your mind

Seventh Tenet

THE REVELATION

I first met Granny in 1969, when I attended the birthday party for the person who eventually became my daughter and the mother of my two grandsons. It was her 8th birthday party and she was having the time of her life. My soon to be daughter was a beautiful little girl with the ability to wrap you around her baby finger in a heartbeat — and she knew it! Not only did she know it, she knew how to use it to her advantage. That's how I became her father!

Now don't get me wrong, I was truly in love with her mother, and we did have a wonderful relationship going on already, but guess who was always the consummate match maker saying things like "Mommy, he's so nice" or "Mommy, I really like him" or "Are you going to marry him mommy?", or "He's so handsome." or "Granny really likes him, too!" You get the picture don't you? So in keeping with the game plan, the wedding took place on Pearl Harbor Day – December 7, 1974 – and that made me a part of Granny's family — or, did it make Granny a part of my family? Whatever...!

Over the next twenty plus years I got to know granny pretty well. She was an older version of my daughter Sabrina — full of vim and vigor, a real spitfire, and always on the go. Believe it or not, granny was still working with special needs children as a volunteer grandmother when she was well into her late eighties. She also had been diagnosed with cancer over 40 years prior to her death. Based on what I've been told, she never had any professional medical treatment for the disease prior to her death at the tender age of 91!

Eva Mae Edwards was born on August 28, 1905 in Fayette, Mississippi. Granny always talked about her "secret home remedies!" She had a remedy for just about anything imaginable — including: insect bites, colds, stiff joints, runny noses, itching eyes, boils, earaches, toothaches, headaches, baldness, stuttering, flatulence, ugliness, and on and on. You name it, and granny had a remedy for it! Well...maybe she didn't have a cure for ugliness, or some of that other stuff—but she was good!

Case in point! I believe it was the summer of 1975 and school had recessed for the summer when we allowed Sabrina to go spend a couple of weeks with granny. When Sabrina left home to go visit granny she had a skin condition that caused an irritable rash in the folds of her neck, arms and leg joints. At one point the rash became so severe she was under the care of a prominent dermatologist in the area who came highly recommended. But, after months of treatment, the eczema persisted. It just wouldn't respond to treatment!

When the two weeks hiatus with granny was about to end, we received a phone call from Sabrina that went something like this, "Hi dad, granny wants me to stay for another week so I can help her in the garden." "Aren't you ready to come home yet?" Her reply, "No, granny wants me to stay a little bit longer; you know how much she loves having me here." "Where's granny now?" "She went to the store, but she told me to tell you it was ok if I stayed. Please tell me it is ok for me to stay— please, please, please!" I told her if it was ok with granny, she could stay. The phone clicked, end of conversation.

I figured something in the milk wasn't clean, but I went along with the program anyway, because Sabrina was the apple of granny's eye, and granny was her saving grace. They were like two peas in a pod. Plus, I had my own motive! No kid, no cartoons, and no clothing restrictions around the house for one more week! Hallelujah!

When my wife Sandra, and I, went to pick Sabrina up the following week it was the usual ritual — she went up and down the street saying goodbyes to her little friends while the two of us visited with granny. Initially, we didn't notice anything different when Sabrina got into the car, but shortly after we got back home as Sandra was examining her to see if the eczema had spread to any other area of her body she discovered something that took us both by surprise! There was no evidence of the eczema anywhere on her person! Not on her neck, arms, legs — nothing, not a trace! We both exclaimed in unison "What happened?"

Sabrina said "granny kept rubbing some sticky stuff on me that she made out of apples, or something." Sabrina couldn't tell us exactly what it was that granny had applied to her skin. All she would say is that it smelled like fruit. Sandra phoned granny immediately and asked her what did she use to eradicate the eczema? Granny told her it was an old remedy she had concocted from apple peels a long time ago — she wouldn't reveal the remaining ingredients, all she would do was chuckle. That was well over forty years ago and to this day— Sabrina has never had even a trace of eczema! As Sandra was speaking to granny, Sabrina was in the background chiming in, "don't forget she cured my "pink eye" in one day — remember mommy, remember? Granny's always curing me!"

Granny was amazing! I can remember visiting her one Sunday afternoon shortly after the New Year in 1987. I was still smoking cigarettes at the time. I was puffing on two or three packs of menthols a day! So here I was sitting at the dining room table, smoking, hacking, and coughing every now and then. Granny was puttering around in her small kitchen cooking up a mess of collard greens and southern fried chicken, as part of the Sunday feast we were anxiously awaiting.

It was above the din of the clinking and clanging pots and pans that I heard her soft voice say, "Ricky, you know you need to quit smoking those things— don't you?" And that was all she said. Again, "You need to quit smoking those things!" I acknowledged her wisdom and told her I wished I could quit, but hadn't been successful in my prior attempts at cessation. Granny said, "If you are serious about quitting — I can tell you how to do it."

To be honest, I really wasn't interested in quitting at the time, because I enjoyed puffing on those lung burners! Sound familiar? I lied and told her I was serious about wanting to kick the habit. Yes, I lied! Shame on me! In any event, granny took a seat beside me at the small table and told me the following story:

She said when she was a young girl growing up in rural Mississippi where a lot of folks had a penchant for using tobacco and alcohol. Granny indicated that she had developed the habit of smoking cigarettes and dipping snuff. She laughed, and said she could spit tobacco juice with the best of them. She also admitted to taking a sip of "moonshine" every now and again. Granny said she would sneak into the "Juke Joint" and have the time of her life! Mind you, she was only 15 years old at the time.

Granny told me she had left the juke joint one Saturday night alone, and had to walk about two miles down the road to her house. She said she was within eyesight of her house when a bright light suddenly illuminated the road ahead of her. Granny said the hair on the nape of her neck stood up! Then to her amazement she said a little old white man appeared in the middle of the road in the midst of the light. At this point my ears perked up a bit, because I hadn't anticipated such a story— but this really piqued my curiosity! I thought she was going to tell me to drink a cup of cow pie tea, or some other gross tasting remedy that she had concocted in her small kitchen — but that was far from the case! "Tap the person next to you, and say E.T. phone home!"

Granny went on to say the little old white man told her not be afraid, because he wasn't there to harm her. She said, the man admonished her about defiling her body with tobacco and alcohol. He told her that smoking cigarettes and dipping snuff would injure her mouth and lungs, and drinking alcohol would injure her liver: But not to worry because he would tell her what to do to divest herself from those enemies of her body.

She said the little white man told her that her body was Gods Temple and he would give her a blessing that would transform her life forever if she would only follow his instructions. Granny said he went on to say that once she had received this blessing she would be able to bestow the same blessing on to others seeking wisdom. All they had to do was believe. Granny said she followed everything the man had told her to do, and lo and behold it worked! She said when she put the man's instructions to the test she no longer had any desire to smoke, dip snuff, or drink alcohol any time after that day, or for the rest of her life! "Now, I'm really listening!

Here's what she told me and instructed me to do. She said, "Ricky, if you want to rid yourself of that nasty habit you can do it. But you can only do it on the 13th day of the month! The 13th day of any month you choose is the day you can divest yourself of your habit." Granny also told me not to smoke after midnight on the 12th day of the month I choose to quit— and I was not to smoke all day on the 13th of that same month. She told me if I followed her advice, when I awake on the 14th day of that month, I would not want to smoke another cigarette in my life!

Granny also warned me not to cheat and smoke a cigarette on the 13th— because by taking just one puff on the 13th the blessing would fail— and I would have to wait until the 13th day of the following month to try it again! If this predicament should befall you, reread the Sixth Tenet and follow the advice therein, and you will be fine until the 13th day of the following month. <u>Do not smoke on the 13th of the month!</u>

Granny went on to say, if I followed her instructions I would be successful and then I too could pass the blessing on to others who may be struggling with an addiction or any other habit they may want to rid themselves of. The 13th day of the month is the key! I told you it was unbelievable, didn't I? Open your mind! You can quit smoking in just ONE day — 24 hours! Believe me!

The 13th of January rolled around so fast I was puffing away before I realized I had goofed up my drop-dead day! Now I must wait until the following month. As I stated in the Introduction of this book, my grandson Terrance was due to arrive on this earth sometime in early April, and as a result, I decided his birth would give me incentive to quit. I told myself, February 12th would be the last time a cigarette would touch my lips. However, I did take advantage of my mistake and continued to puff away until February 12th. *"Smoke, smoke, smoke that cigarette: Smoke, smoke, smoke yourself to death!"*

Finally, February 12, 1987 rolled around! It wasn't a welcomed day, because during the entire month of January all I could think about was how many cigarettes I would normally smoke along with my morning coffee. How many I would smoke when I had the occasional cocktail. How many I would usually smoke on the golf course, and how many I smoked just because I had them.

It was if I was about to lose my best friend. The thought of quitting frightened me — I figured if this worked like granny said it would, I'm going to be one miserable so and so! Although I was still a little skeptical I did just as Granny had instructed me to do. I sucked it up and got on with it! "I'm the man, baby — let's get it on!" "Okay, okay I didn't say so and so — you know what I said!"

I fought the urge to light up on February 13th although I wanted to smoke in the worst way! Imagine — a three pack a day, coffee drinking, chain smoking knucklehead trying not to smoke all day long! The deep breathing exercise that granny taught me really came to the rescue though. <u>When the urge to give up and light up overwhelmed me, I did the exercise — eventually the nicotine graving would diminish as Granny promised it would. It was tough, but I managed to stick it out until bedtime. I was determined not to fail!</u>

When I awoke on February 14th I went about my normal daily routine. Turned on the television, made coffee, retrieved the newspaper, did my toiletries, made a quick snack, ate, showered, dressed, and before

I knew it I was at work! Not once did I think about a cigarette! I had eaten breakfast, which included my morning coffee, and I never thought about lighting up! Normally I would smoke two or three cigarettes with my breakfast! I went the entire day and never thought about smoking a single cigarette! That was over twenty five years ago, and I have never touched nor craved another cigarette since that day!

When I asked granny what happened to the little old white man in the road, she told me he had disappeared just as he had appeared — in a flash of light! Okay, now don't shoot the messenger like my friend from Ohio. I'm just sharing what I was told. This is granny's version of what happened, not mine! However, there is one aspect of granny's story I wish I had been more inquisitive about, and that's the description of the "little old white man" she alluded to, but I guess that will remain a mystery.

Eighth Tenet

BELIEVE IN YOU

I was in my library attempting to put the finishing touches on this book when I received a telephone call from Judie, a friend of the family inquiring about the well-being of our daughter, who was battling a serious health challenge at the time — she wanted to wish Sabrina well.

During our conversation I asked her if she was still bowling, or had she finally given it up. She told me she was still active in her weekly bowling league and enjoying it! I didn't ask about her average, because I assumed it probably was still 137! You see, we used to bowl in the same coed bowling league at one time, and her average plateaued at 137. Year after year 137 — never more, never less, 137 was it! My sister-in-law Pat still bowls in a league with her, and from time to time I would inquire about my friends average — the answer was always the same, 137! So I assumed it must still be 137 to this day!

I guess you're wondering what makes this story relevant with smoking cessation — right? Put it this way — I assumed Judie's bowling average was still 137, although I didn't have any proof for such an assumption. I also assumed she was still a heavy smoker, because when we bowled together in the same league, she smoked like a chimney! When I asked her if she was still a heavy smoker like in the past, I wasn't expecting the answer she gave me. She said she had quit! Now, I wasn't shocked that she had actually quit — but it was how she went about it — hence the relevance of this story.

Judie is currently a member of a weekly bid whist club, of which my sister-in-law Brenda is also a member, and it was during one of their weekly card playing sessions that Judie complained of her inability to quit smoking. Although she had managed to cut down to only a couple of cigarettes a day—she couldn't close the deal. She said that's when my sister-in-law told her to try what I had shared with some of the guests who attended a cookout she hosted at her home one summer.

Judie said Brenda told her about granny's revelation, and how various people had quit smoking because of it. Judie decided because the 13th of the month was close to her birthday she would make quitting smoking a birthday present to herself. She informed me that she followed what was revealed to her and quit COLD TURKEY overnight! I almost dropped the telephone when I heard that!

When Judie told me she had quit smoking cigarettes over ten years ago, I wanted to know how she came to quit. What motivated her to quit smoking cigarettes after all those years of being addicted? She said she decided to try to quit one more time, as she put it, because she was drinking too much coffee, and smoking too many cigarettes! She surmised if she could give up drinking coffee, she probably could quit smoking cigarettes also, because she had the tendency to morph into a chain smoker whenever she drank coffee. Does her story sound familiar?

When I informed Judie about the book I was writing concerning granny's revelation and how it has helped so many people quit smoking, she asked me to please include her story, because she wanted everyone to know when you believe you can achieve a given thing — you can! Judie was finally really ready to quit, and she did!

In the third tenet I wrote about speaking to a congregation associated with the chaplaincy program in place at various Big Three facilities located throughout the United States. When I was introduced to the assembly, my friend Leon told the group I had virtually saved his life, because of what I told him about granny during our walk in Washington D.C.

There was just one little flaw in the introduction though: He gave the group some erroneous information concerning granny's revelation. He told the assembly a little alien in a white suit, gave granny the power to bless people, so they could quit bad habits. What she actually said was what I shared with you in this book, and there is no mention of a little dude in a white suit running around giving out blessings. Read the Seventh tenet again.

After making the necessary corrections to the story, I spoke about the need to believe in self. I said maybe our success had nothing to do with granny's revelation at all — but just <u>believing</u> that it did might have guaranteed our success! Believe in yourself and you too will be successful. Think positive, and positive results will emanate.

Granny overcame, because she believed what the little man told her. I overcame, because I believed what granny told me. The folks I wrote about in the various tenets overcame, because they believed what was revealed to them. You too will also overcome if you believe what I have shared with you. If you can conceive it and believe it— you can achieve it!

Well, there you have it. Now that you have finished reading this book up to this point, I sincerely hope you take advantage of knowing you now possess the where-with-all to successfully emancipate yourself from your addiction to smoking or any other form of nicotine addiction that may be plaguing you. It's entirely up to you. So quit blowing smoke and get on with it!

God bless and good luck!

About the Author

Richard H. Bobo said he wrote this book, because so many people asked him to write it. Prior to his retirement in 2004, he worked as an Administrative Assistant to the President of the United Automobile Workers (UAW). And over the years during his travels, he shared granny's story with hundreds of people who successfully kicked the habit COLD TURKEY. You will read several of their testimonials interlaced within various tenets throughout this book.

Twenty eight years ago Mr. Bobo smoked nearly three packs of cigarettes a day, and was a severely addicted chain smoker, lighting one up after another. But today he is completely free of that debilitating habit, because he learned how to quit smoking cigarettes COLD TURKEY in ONE day!

Mr. Bobo's decision to quit smoking cigarettes in 1987 has played a big part in him being around today, to see the birth of his great granddaughter — his grandson's baby girl! That's right: today he's a great grandpa and there's STILL no secondhand smoke in the house!

Symbolic Meaning of 13

*G*ranny was adamant about me quitting smoking on the 13th of the month, and no other date, lest I would fail: which leads me to believe the "little old white man," gave her more information about the number 13, and it's prominence in our everyday lives than she shared with me. How did she know I would fail, had he not explained to her why SHE would fail? The influence of the number 13 and its relevance is all around us and we don't even realize it! I am so grateful that I was enlightened and made aware of that fact!

The number 13 is not an unfortunate number, as is generally supposed. It is clearly evident that 13 is the most glorified number of the United States of America. The phrase "July the Fourth" contains 13 letters and the number 4 (1+3), the birth date number of the United States (July 4, 1776), which leads us to the real reason why the "founding fathers" chose this date as the official birth date of the United States of America. Starting with the 13 colonies, the first national flag had 13 stars, and even today it still has 13 horizontal stripes: 6 white and 7 red. On the reverse side of the $1.00 bill there are 13 levels on the pyramid of the Great Seal. The two words above the pyramid, which reads "Annuit Coeptis" consists of 13 letters; the eagle on the right side is holding a banner in its beak that bears the motto "E pluribus Unum," which contains 13 letters. The eagle has 13 tail feathers, and on its breast there is a shield with 13 vertical stripes. The eagle also holds an olive branch with 13 leaves and

13 berries in its right talon, and 13 arrows in its left. Over the eagle's head are 13 stars that form the six-pointed "Star of David." You should really think about this one, because it could save you a bunch of dough! The average 1 pack a day smoker could possibly save over $2000.00 a year by opting to quit smoking. Some folks could save even more, as cigarette prices tend to vary from state to state, and costing anywhere from $5.00 a pack in West Virginia to almost $12.00 a pack in New York. That's a lot of cash going up in smoke: Unless you've got money to burn! Tap somebody and say, "He just couldn't resist saying that!"

Taylor Swift, the singer songwriter was born on December 13th, and considers 13 her lucky number, because of the lucky events happening when that number appears. Her debut album went gold in 13 weeks, and being seated at award shows in the 13th seat, row, or section good things abound. She also has the number 13 written on her hand when she performs at concerts. So once again, as you can see, the number 13 is not an unfortunate number, as is generally supposed. It has become so firmly associated in the popular mind with the notion of "bad luck" that it is easy to forget the fact that in the ancient mystic religions 13 was the characteristic number of participants in many orders and groups, including sacred meals – a fact reflected in the size of the original Nazarene Last Supper. The number 13 is also the most fortunate number for Africans, African-Americans, and people the world over of African descent. It was venerated in ancient Egypt from time immemorial, and was held in great reverence by the ancient Egyptians. The 13th Amendment of the United States Constitution Officially Abolished Slavery and Involuntary Servitude, except for Punishment for a Crime. Apparitions of the Virgin of Fatima in 1917 were claimed to appear on the 13th day of the month for six consecutive months.

It takes 13 days to change from Full Moon to New Moon, and 13 days to move back; with 1 day Full and 1 day New to equal 28 days of the Lunar Cycle. The average celestial motion of the Moon is 13° per day, and 13 weeks is the time it takes the earth to travel from the equinoxes to the solstices. It takes the earth 13 weeks to travel from the first day of spring (March 20th) to the first day of summer (June 21st); 13 weeks from the first day of summer to the first day of fall (Sept. 23rd); 13 weeks from the first day of fall to the first day of winter (Dec. 21st); and it takes the earth 13 weeks to travel from the first day of winter to the first day of spring... (13x4=52) which is the time it takes (in weeks) the earth to make one complete revolution around the Sun, and in most years lunation's occur 13 times. The fear of the number 13 is unfounded internationally as well. It is an honored number in many countries throughout the world. There are 13 occurrences of the quantity 13 in the design of the Great Pyramid of Giza in Egypt, the largest stone edifice ever built. In the Indian Pantheon there are 13 Buddha's. The mystical discs that surmount Indian and Chinese pagodas are 13 in number. Enshrined in the Temple of Atsuta in Japan is a sacred sword with 13 objects of mystery forming its hilt. And 13 was the sacred number of the ancient Aztec's, who had 13 snake gods. The 13th letter of the English alphabet is M, which finds its roots in the 13th letter of the Hebrew alphabet, "mem" (meaning mother), which was the ancient Phoenician word for water. The ancient Egyptian word for water was "moo." M is the most sacred of all the letters, for it symbolizes water, where all life began. It is the root of the word "mother," and relates to the evolutionary destiny of Africans, African-Americans, and all people of African descent who are ruled by the number 13. Additional information on this subject can be found on the Internet.

Printed in the United States
By Bookmasters